THE CAUCASIAN BOOK
OF LONGEVITY AND WELL-BEING

THE CAUCASIAN BOOK
OF LONGEVITY AND WELL-BEING

Murat Yagan

Threshold Books

Threshold Books is committed to publishing books of spiritual significance and high literary quality. All Threshold Books have sewn bindings and are printed on acid-free paper.

We will be happy to send you a catalog.
Threshold Books, RD4, Box 600, Putney, Vermont 05346

Illustrations courtesy of Planeta Publishers, Progress Publishers, National Geographic.

Copyright © 1988, all rights reserved.

Library of Congress Catalog Card Number 88-040222
ISBN 0-939660-28-8

Library of Congress Cataloging-in-Publication Data:

Yagan, Murat.
        The Caucasian book of longevity and well-being.

        1. Longevity. 2. Abkhasians--Health and hygiene.
I. Title.
RA776.75.Y34   1988   613   88-40222
ISBN 0-939660-28-8

CONTENTS

7
Preface

11
Introduction
Who We Are

13
Chapter One
Physical Man

31
Chapter Two
Psychological Man

35
Chapter Three
Ecological Man

57
Chapter Four
Man as a Whole

PREFACE

This book is about more than simply living a long life. It considers the quality of life that the long-lived tribes of the Caucasus, especially the Abkhasians, enjoy. It is more than diet, more than skin brushing, more than exercising, more than humor that enables Abkhasians to live long and satisfying lives. It is a combination of these ingredients plus customs unknown to North Americans that makes life a long and healthy prospect for these people.

Few know the customs and traditions of the Abkhasian people from the inside out. Although books have been written about the beauty and mystery and the life of the Caucasus, they have all been written by observers of the tradition. Here is a statement by one who was born into it and who lives it.

The ancestral line of Murat Yagan originates in Abkhasia, in an area between the northeast shores of the Black Sea and the main range of the Caucasus Mountains. Abkhasia is protected from bitter northern winds by the mountains and tempered by the warm, humid breezes from the Black Sea; the climate is mild, the landscape rugged and lush. Murat Yagan's ancestors were a warrior-trained, well-disciplined mountain people whose roots can be traced back at least 26,000 years—some believe to the origins of the human race. Abkhasian longevity is legendary: it is not unusual for men and women alike to live full and productive lives past their 125th year. Murat Yagan belongs to the ruling class of noblemen in his tribe. He is the chief of the tribe, as were his father and his grandfather before him.

According to Abkhasian tradition, to be a nobleman meant to be at the beck and call of the tribe at all times. The Abkhasian nobility was totally dedicated and responsive to the well-being of the other members of the tribe, caring for and protecting them, and providing for them a source of direction and courage. The rulers were the servants of the tribe, and anyone could claim the rulers' time—even in the middle of the night, if he so desired; even if all he wanted was to share a glass of wine.

This tribal society adored its leaders. The leader was all, and a leader was appointed for each event, be it a picnic or a battle. One submitted to the will of the leader fearlessly and confidently, for no one doubted that the leader had the best interests of his people at heart. So conditioned were they to this way of being that hesitation or lack of submission seldom occurred. So much love and respect was exchanged among the various "classes" within the tribes that their unity made them nearly unbeatable in battles or competitions. No one in the Abkhasian tradition was ever really lonely. He might spend time alone, but he never felt himself to be "by himself." If he wasn't surrounded by friends or work partners or family, then his ancestors, those who formed his genetic line, were with him.

The office of tribal chief was not specifically passed down from father to son, but was invited on the basis of merit as well as heredity. The Abkhasian idea of aristocracy meant that one found his place in society based on his inherited genetic characteristics. These characteristics were not only simple physical attributes, nor were they restricted to talents such as an ability in music or sport. The Abkhasian tradition stated that one inherited his tendencies and capacities in the spiritual realms as well. Thus everyone had his place based on his hereditary line. Although this might seem static and even unfair to the North American mind, nothing could be farther from the truth. These people pulled their weight evenly in their tribes. No one was thought of as "less than" because he wasn't part of the ruling class. Each class had its field of expertise, and each position was totally respected by the entire tribe. The serf was as much beloved and respected by the nobleman as was the nobleman by the serf. Each was aware of how much he needed the other and each depended on the other, certain that the other would do his job thoroughly and precisely.

Murat Yagan tells the story of Daruk, a 208-year-old coachman in Murat's childhood Istanbul house. Daruk belonged to the class of serf. When Murat's teenage aunts wanted to go out and enjoy the performance of a visiting European theatre or musical troop, they had to ask Murat's father, Met, for permission. Sometimes as many as eight girls had to find a way through Met's door. He worked as

Preface 9

a politician in the Turkish government and was often inaccessible because he was tied up with affairs of state or tribe. If it seemed inappropriate for the girls to approach Met personally, they would find Daruk and ask his permission. They knew that whatever Daruk asked would not be refused.

Just after the Bolshevik Revolution, Murat Yagan's grandfather led a group of 15,000 Abkhasians out of the mountains and down into Turkey. There, many of them maintained their customs and traditions, gathering together in villages populated only by members of the tribe. Some, such as Murat's father, settled in Istanbul. Although many from the Caucasus became "Turkified," many of the old customs remain to this day. It is said that one can always tell when a man or woman from the Caucasus walks down the street. He or she looks neither to the right nor the left, but above the heads of everyone. If there are two walking abreast, heaven help anyone else on the sidewalk. If more room is needed, one simply has to give way to the Abkhasian, for he doesn't see you.

Murat Yagan's life has led him from the Caucasus to Turkey and finally to Canada. He lives without pretense or fanfare, making his living as a carpenter and travelling around British Columbia wherever his work takes him. He has long abandoned the title of chief of his tribe, but his house remains open to the people of his tradition; hospitality is a mainstay of the traditional Abkhasian home life. At this writing, Murat is 71 years old and in excellent health. Not many teenagers can keep up with him!

This book, then, is a first-hand statement of the holistic health practices which are followed by the Abkhasian people. They care for their minds, bodies, spirits, and emotions in the same way that they care for each other. Full unity is theirs, within and without. And that is what makes it possiblefor them not only to lead long lives, but also to create and enjoy the quality of their lives. Here is how they do it.

February 1988

Joan McIntyre
Vernon, British Columbia

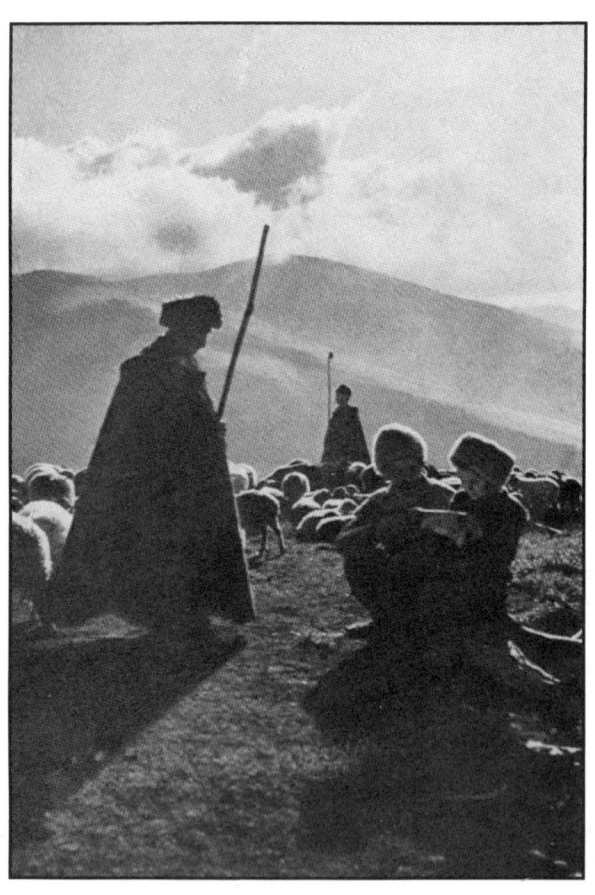

WHO WE ARE

After having emigrated from my native country, Abkhasia, on the Black Sea slopes of the Caucasian Mountains, after the Bolshevik Revolution (1918), in my very early childhood, I have been in eighteen different countries for various lengths of time, until eventually I made my home in Canada in 1963, at the age of forty-seven.

In every country I have been, when people came to know that I was an Abkhasian, they would have one thing common to say: "Hey, tell me the secret of the commonly known longevity of Abkhasians." "We heard they eat a lot of yogurt, is that it?"—"We heard they had the practice of brushing their skin all over every day, is that it?"—"We heard about the extraordinarily favorable climate in the mountains, is that it?"—"We heard about their peculiar concept of sexuality, is that it?"

Well, I wish it was that simple. The answer is very clear and concrete, but not simple.

To live long, it is not necessary to be Abkhasian by race, but it is necessary to grasp their traditional discipline of living and the philosophy behind it. That very thing shall be found in this book in its fullness, but how much of it every reader will get, I do not know, and I make no guarantees, as every Abkhasian does not live following the tradition of the ancients and therefore does not live long.

The name of the game is *discipline*.

Before we start dealing with any *thing* in general, we have to know about this *thing* as much as we can—its entity, its identity, its characteristics, its nature and the physical, chemical and social—in other words, Cosmic—laws it complies with.

Every living entity exists and functions on five levels: Physical, Intellectual, Spiritual, Psychic, and Ecological. The intellectual, spiritual and psychic levels together constitute the mind; all three of them we can sum up under the name "psychological." The psychological levels represent, respectively, various levels of subtlety of mind; just as ice, liquid and vapor represent various levels of subtlety of water, for example.

To conduct a comprehensive study, we consider the Human in its five functional levels and not only in one, such as for example the physical, although our subject being longevity it may seem that our studies should be in the physical matters, namely anatomical and physiological. In other words, we consider the Human in its holistic sense of being. All the five functions should work simultaneously and in full coordination.

Here, I shall take in hand each functional level, one by one, and I shall relate what Abkhasian elders say from their ancient wisdom about each functional level. Many things that Abkhasian wisdom professes may not fit today's medical, hygienic and psychological concepts, but after all, it was those ancient, maybe half-savage and ignorant people who achieved the kind of longevity we are talking about today in our hopelessly sophisticated era.

Chapter One
PHYSICAL MAN

The food that the human body needs to perpetuate its physical existence is taken in eating, drinking, and breathing.

EATING

The whole of the food taken in through this way is not utilized for the sustenance of the body. Food is digested and assimilated; the sustaining part is used by the body and the remnant is rejected; we shall call it primary refuse. The sustaining part which is kept in, while being utilized by the body's metabolism, produces another secondary residual matter which, if not rejected, accumulates in the physical system in the form of toxins, and needs special treatment to be gotten rid of. This toxin, which we shall call secondary refuse, accumulates in the mucus that covers the membranes of internal organs to moisten and protect them. The mucus, although indispensable for the function it exercises, is unnecessary and harmful when produced in excess. But, as more toxins accumulate in it, more mucus is produced to harbor them, and if the necessary actions are not taken to purge the body of the toxins, they have a poisonous effect on tissues and cause antibody formations. The malfunction of the whole system becomes inevitable, as does the inefficiency of all five functional levels. The accumulation of toxins may finally, in the long run, lead to cancerous developments. *This is, at its least, one fundamental factor which curtails human longevity.*

Some kinds of food are more likely to produce this residual matter, or toxin, and some are less likely. Toxin, being a colloidal proteinaceous substance, is more likely to be produced by foods rich in protein. But the human body needs protein. So, the solution of the problem does not lie in avoiding eating protein, but lies in paying special care to eliminating the toxin produced. So, here comes one fundamental statement:

RULE 1
It is not so much the question of what to eat, but rather how to eat.

By "how" I mean all aspects of how to prepare the food, how frequently to eat, when to eat, how much to eat, and what rules to follow.

Some think that by following a strictly vegetarian diet one can secure longevity. There are a lot of loopholes in this thinking. It is true that a vegetarian diet produces fewer toxins, especially when the food is prepared in the correct manner of cooking or not cooked at all; still, a vegetarian diet is not totally toxin-free. The same elimination of the accumulated toxins is necessary. And, on the other hand, the human digestive system is not made, as some of today's Western dietitians think, to be specifically vegetarian, but omnivorous. Any animal system put together by nature to be strictly vegetarian (herbivorous) cannot be converted into being carnivorous, and vice-versa. No matter how much a horse is starving, you cannot put a piece of steak in front of it and make it eat. The system of some animals, such as rats, pigs, and bears, is made adaptable to both diets by nature, and the human being is one such animal.

Elimination of the toxins and consequently elimination of the excess of mucus in the system is taken care of by nature, in wild life, under circumstantial conditions. First, let me explain the procedure of eliminating toxins.

When the food is taken in, assimilation starts in the stomach, continues in the small intestines and finally, with very little intensity, finishes in the colon. After digestion is completed in the stomach, while the assimilation is still in process, nature starts its cleaning job in the stomach and continues it in the intestines. The stomach secretions have finished their function of attacking the food and decomposing it into assimilable matter. What is not useful is cleaned away, as well as remnants of refuse which may be left behind in the system. When the stomach is performing this cleaning job, certain chemical reactions take place, as well as physical activities such as peristaltic movements of the stomach and intestines. All these activities create a sensation very similar to hunger, and the individual feels like eating. This is a fictitious, deceptive hunger; it will pass away in a very short period of time if ignored. Nature will complete its cleaning job and then a second and more durable feeling of hunger will prevail. It is also recommended that this be ignored and that one wait until the third surge of hunger, which will be the real one, indeed. So that is how nature takes care of the elimination of toxins and consequently of excess mucus, if given a chance.

For carnivorous animals with protein-rich diets, the accumulation of toxin and production of excess mucus is greater than for herbivorous animals with light diets.

In wild life, nature takes care of granting to the digestive system the chance of dealing with toxins through circumstantial conditions. Let us take the example of tigers or wolves. Because of the risks, hazards, perils and tiresome labor of hunting for their game, they procrastinate until they get helplessly hungry. Then they set off on the venture of hunting. They spend some time in the hit or miss process until they get hold of a meal. When they have it, they eat their very fill until they fall asleep on their backs. They do not eat again for at least three to four days, during which time their system is completely purified from toxins.

Herbivorous animals graze all day long, never really getting full; they stop only when they get tired and sleepy, because what they eat does not have substance enough to sustain the animal without eating for three or four days. The accumulation of toxins is not very substantial, but it is there. But because their food supply is dependent on seasons, their digestive system is subjected to seasonal, circumstantial rest, during which the system has a chance for elimination of toxins.

For some animals with a mixed diet, what is called hibernation is a wise method of nature.

Because animals do not have willpower and reason to resist the temptation of desire, they are taken care of by nature; domestic animals, which are at the mercy of the foolishness of Man, do not have the same chance; therefore their longevity is curtailed.

To achieve the same results afforded by nature to wild animals, we human beings have to discipline ourselves according to the wisdom of our knowledge through willpower and reason, because the circumstantial conditions of nature do not exist to control the temptation of our desires. All we have to do is to put a long interval of time between any two meals. This interval of time is determined according to the kind of food we take in—a longer interval in the case of a carnivorous diet and a shorter one in the case of a vegetarian diet. And more importantly, no nibbling at all in the meantime.

In light of the explanation I have given so far, it is obvious that we should be as concerned with how completely and properly our system gets rid of refuse of all kinds as we should be with what and how we eat.

Let us stop for a moment now, and observe ourselves as today's Westerners. Let us be sensible: How far away are we from the true diet, just as much of it as we understand so far? First of all, we were driven in the wrong direction by medical advisors. For decades and decades it was considered healthier to eat a little at a time and to eat more frequently. So, as a common North American, we get up in the morning and have breakfast—bacon and eggs, maybe, with at least a couple of cups of coffee. A couple of hours later we stop for a coffee break, a doughnut or two and a couple of cups of coffee—not uncommon. A couple of hours later, lunch-break—sandwiches and coffee. A couple of hours later, coffee break, with coffee, cookies or sandwiches again. Two or three hours later, a substantial supper—steaks, or stew, potatoes, and so on. Can anybody tell me what kind of chance we are giving for the elimination of refuse and the purification of toxins? And the only thing people ask is: "What do Abkhasians eat to live long?" Nobody asks, "What do they do to keep their systems pure and free of refuse?"

Physical Man

Abkhasians do not eat anything particularly and noticeably different from what we eat here in North America. But they pay particular attention to how to eat and how to rid their systems of refuse of all kinds. We shall come to that in detail later. Now, it is enough to state:

RULE 2
It is important not only what and how to eat, but also how to eliminate the residual refuse resultant from eating.

DRINKING

Some liquid is taken in from the water content of what is eaten, and some is taken in from direct drinking of liquid. How much liquid will be drunk in liquid form depends on one's eating diet. The one who follows a vegetarian diet mostly in green form will supplement the water supply with direct drinking less than the one who follows a meat or dry diet, such as a diet of nuts and cereals. Drinking is very important, especially when the system is involved in its toxin cleaning process. We shall cover this topic when dealing with *elimination of refuse*.

Alcoholic beverages should only be taken in moderation and preferably with meals, and people who follow a vegetarian diet should exercise moderation even more scrupulously. Exercising right drinking at the right time with the right food is as important as right eating. So we can state:

RULE 3
Drinking right is as important as eating right.

BREATHING

Breathing is the most important factor of physical life. Life starts with breathing. According to Abkhasian spiritual teaching, the fetus becomes a living entity upon receiving the first breath. Before breathing, it is a living thing, a potential human entity, but not an independent living entity. Note the difference between a living thing and a living entity. According to what is reported from life experiences, a man can live forty-one days without eating, five days without drinking, but only five minutes without breathing.

As a result of being alive, a burning phenomenon takes place in the tissues, the residue of which is carbon. Red hemoglobin, floating in the blood and carrying oxygen acquired from the breath, visits this carbon, which unites with the oxygen forming carbon dioxide which is exhaled by the breath.

Our respiratory system can work in two ways: consciously and unconsciously. Without being conscious of it, we keep breathing all day, in every single moment of our lives, normally fourteen times a minute. But also we can breathe consciously, increasing or decreasing the length or frequency of our breath, for health reasons and also in certain kinds of intellectual, spiritual, psychic or, in one word, psychological exercises. The working and the efficiency of our mental system is related to the health and well-being of our nervous system, which is the home of our mind; and the well-being of our nervous system is related to its being free from toxins. The nerves themselves may be buried in an excess of fat, mucus, and consequently, of toxins, as a result of inefficient elimination of residual refuse. The nervous system then loses its sharpness of functioning as a home for the mind. And what we call *clarity of mind* dwindles just because the supply of oxygen to take away carbon from the tissues in the form of carbon dioxide slows down. It becomes a difficult process instead of being a smooth-running process as it would be in the case of a toxin-free system. So, it becomes obvious that our mental health is subject to elimination of toxins like the rest of our system. We shall come back to the effects of breathing on our well-being later on when we talk about Man as a Whole. For now, it suffices to say:

RULE 4
The efficiency of our breathing is dependent on a toxin-free system.

ELIMINATION OF REFUSE

Primary Refuse

What we have called the primary refuse is produced as a result of metabolism taking place in the whole body and is the unutilizable remnants of food. Primary refuse appears in five forms: excrement, urine, sweat, carbon dioxide, and uninseminated ovum (in the case of women).

Secondary Refuse

All the forms of primary refuse have to be eliminated from the body, and they are, but never absolutely one hundred per cent at once. There is always some remnant left behind for the system to throughly purge. This remnant which needs further purging we have called secondary refuse.

This secondary refuse appears, in the various places in the system, in five forms: toxin, mucus, fat, stones, and cholesterol. The forms of secondary refuse are accumulations of unnecessary matter in the system. Although they appear as five distinctly independent forms, all of them are engendered by the existence of toxin in the system, which causes malfunctioning of the human machinery in every corner of the body (except in special pathological cases, in which there might be some other causes). In other words, if necessary treatment for elimination of toxin is successfully exercised in the first place, the formation of all the rest of these secondary refuses would be unlikely. I am going to deal with all these refuses one by one and relate how Abkhasians help the body to eliminate them.

Toxin

Toxin, roughly speaking, is simply an unused protein left behind in a colloidal form, which makes its home in the mucus on the membranes of every tissue and especially in the digestive system. As I explained previously, the body is capable of getting rid of toxin, if given a chance, which means leaving the body alone in handling the cleaning job during and after assimilation of food, by not disturbing it and introducing untimely food to the system. A traditional Abkhasian eats *one meal a day*. Meat being an important part of the Abkhasian diet, giving this much time to the system was necessary.

Certain recommendations provide further help to the elimination job of the body. It is important to keep physically active, and to have fresh air at least for a couple of hours every day. For people on a meat diet, taking alcoholic beverages with the meal is recommended provided the beverages are naturally fermented drink like wine of all kinds, but not brewed or distilled drink.

Four hours after a meal, when the cleaning job of the system is in full process, a glass of water or of drinks containing bacteria which attack toxin, such as natural, fresh grape juice or yogurt drink—which is called AYRAN and is obtained by beating yogurt and diluting it to the consistency of milk—should be taken. But the yogurt should be a natural home-made yogurt without chemical additives at all, preferably made of non-pasteurized farm milk. Another recommendable drink to disturb and eliminate mucus is an apple cider vinegar drink which is made by mixing in one water glass one tablespoonful of honey, one third of a teacup of apple cider vinegar, and water to fill the glass.

People on a cooked vegetarian diet, including those on a dry-crop diet of foods such as nuts, cereals, and beans, should eat two meals a day, one in the morning and one in the evening. People on a raw green vegetable and fruit diet should eat four meals a day. In both cases, the above mentioned drinks in between meals are recommended.

Mucus

Excess mucus will be eliminated with the elimination of toxin, because excess mucus in the system is the result of the accumulation of toxin. Hot green peppers, taken with meals, are another item to include in the diet to fight against mucus.

Fat

Fat will also be eliminated by following the same discipline, with an exception in the case of individuals who are more prone to accumulate fat. Here, more emphasis should be placed on physical exercise. But eliminating fat should never be achieved by cutting down the food more than it is described above.

Stones

There is little likelihood for the formation of gall bladder or kidney stones when the body is kept reasonably toxin-free. One single preventive is the liquid obtained by drying yogurt. Natural homemade yogurt, made from natural farm milk without using any chemical additives for solidifying or preserving purposes, contains a liquid, light green in color, which can be very easily separated by putting yogurt in a light fabric bag and filtering it. One third of a glass of the liquid can be drunk at a time, three times a day; again, between meals but not with meals.

Cholesterol

Cholesterol is formed in the system and is present in cells and body fluids. Although it is important in physiological processes, cholesterol is harmful when present in excess and causes the hardening of arterial walls (arterio-sclerosis). The excess has to be eliminated and rejected from the system, and it is rejected in excrement, urine and sweat. Further activation is secured by following a toxin-free diet.

But there is one aspect of this particular item which requires further consideration. The portion of cholesterol which is rejected by sweat accumulates on the surface of the skin, covering the pores of the skin and impeding cutaneous respiration. This is where the proverbial skin care of Abkhasians comes from. A traditional Abkhasian who has a fair amount of self-respect would make himself throughly perspire at least once every other day, either by physical exercise, sportive games, horseback riding, working in the garden, cutting firewood, or in a steam bath. Then while the body is still warm and wet in sweat, he will jump in cold water or take a cold shower, wash the sweat off, and brush his skin all over for five to ten minutes. Because soap leaves a film on the skin, he uses a very fine clay instead, then rinses it away with abundant water. To keep the skin moist and soft, he uses a skin cream made of lanolin. Other than that, he rubs and dry-brushes his skin all over at least once a day, preferably after getting up in the morning. Another thing to mention here is that when in bed to sleep, he does not wear anything. He puts on enough bed covers to keep warm, but sleeps naked.

Before closing this section on physical man, I should mention a few more important facts. Once these toxins are loosened in the process of the cleaning job in the digestive system, because they are poisonous, it is important to flush them out of the system as soon as possible. This is best accomplished by the above-mentioned drinks; otherwise the toxins will be re-ingested in the system, causing discomfort such as nausea, headaches and dizziness.

At the beginning of this chapter, I stated that the whole of the food taken in is not utilized for the sustenance of the body; it is processed through digestion and assimilation; the sustaining part is kept to be used and the remnant is rejected. Now, the body exercises some effort and therefore spends some energy to do this job. The energy spent to digest, assimilate and reject each kind of food is not the same, because some foods are more difficult to handle and some less difficult. The usable part of each kind of food goes to restore the body in order to maintain it in the venture of existing and also to replace this energy spent to handle the food. Therefore, when we evaluate the nutritive value of each food, we should not forget that the amount of sustenance going to replace the energy spent by the system for handling the food should be subtracted from the whole of the usable amount and the remainder is the net value of the supportive element.

It can be very clearly seen that any food which contains more nutritive value per unit compared to another food, but which is more difficult to digest and assimilate, may be less useful as a food, if the eventual usable part happens to be less in the final accounting.

Now we come to one of the most interesting aspects of the longevity achieved by Abkhasians.

Physical Man

Some foods are naturally difficult to digest, but most of them we make difficult to digest by our ways of cooking them, such as pan frying. Many foods which are pleasurably eatable uncooked we eat uncooked, but not all of them. For example, an egg is eatable uncooked, but we cook it. Nuts such as walnuts, hazelnuts, and almonds are eatable uncooked, but we toast them, just as a result of bad habits. We sacrifice health to the pleasure of taste through this bad habit of cooking. Any food which is not eatable as is, we indiscriminately cook. These foods, which are not eatable or very difficult to eat as they are in nature, need to go through a certain process of preparation, but does this have to be necessarily and inevitably cooking? Could not we create other ways of preparing them to make them pleasurably eatable without cooking?

Well, this is the kind of food preparation that Abkhasians created. Unfortunately, for the last four or five hundred years, the original Abkhasian art of food preparation degenerated under Turkish, Persian, Greek, Armenian and Russian influences and only some of the ancient recipes still persist. At the end of this chapter I shall give some of the traditional recipes of Abkhasian food preparation, for those who might be wiser than today's Abkhasians.

There is another ancient good habit Abkhasians have lost lately. In the old days they used to obtain their salt from the sea weeds of the Black Sea. Now they lazily use the salt coming from the salt mines of Siberia, as well as sugar from refineries rather than from their beautiful mountain honey.

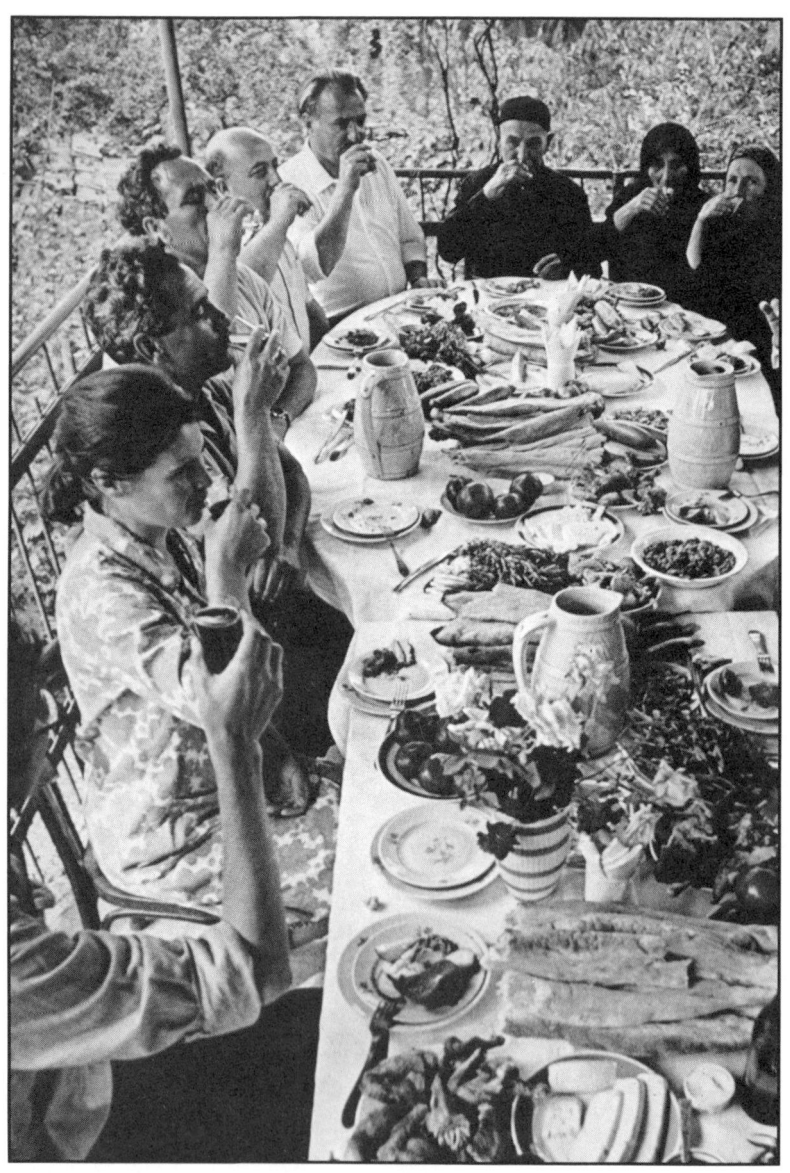

Abkhasians honor their elders at a feast.

TRADITIONAL ABKHASIAN FOOD PREPARATION

Steam Cooking
 The Abkhasian steam cooker is simple. It consists of a covered pot large enough to contain a smaller pan which holds the food to be steamed. Legs on the smaller pan keep the food up above several inches of water in the bottom of the pot. The heated water provides the source of steam.
 The item to be steam-cooked is always cut into small pieces to prevent the outer part from becoming overcooked while the inner part is still uncooked.
 The extent of cooking is always moderate with the food never being overcooked.

Broiling
 Meat is always broiled moderately, only to the extent needed to stop the blood running and cause the redness to fade; an unchangeble habit is always to use fresh meat.
 The fat dripping from meat should never fall on the fire and burn, and the smoke from it be allowed to return to the meat. This is believed to cause cancerous developments. For that purpose a special oven is used. This is an oven of a cylindrical shape, having shelves at either side and a sump at the bottom. The fire is made on the shelves, and pieces of meat are hung in the middle. The heat of the fire hits the meat from the sides and drops of fat fall into the sump and flow away.

Meat Mincing
 Mincing of meat is not recommended to be done in a meat grinder. Meat is minced by cutting with two sharp knives held side by side touching each other cross-wise and moving them simultaneously from left to right in every direction. This way the meat will be minced without suffering any pressure and therefore losing its tasty juice.

TRADITIONAL ABKHASIAN RECIPES

Yogurt

Heat 1 liter milk on medium high heat until it starts rising. Cool it in the same pot for a while. Pour it into a plastic container. Let it cool further, down to body temperature. If it is too warm, yogurt becomes watery and sour; if just at the right temperature, it will be thick and sweet.

Measure two heaping teaspoons of yogurt (your own or commercial) into a teacup; stir in a few tablespoons of milk. Stir this mixture into the milk. Put a lid on the container. Wrap it snugly wih old sweaters. Leave for three or four hours. Take off the lid. Place in the refrigerator and leave for one full day before using.

SAUCES AND DRESSINGS

Purpuljiga (Seasoning Sauce)
1 dozen Mexican hot red peppers (dried)
3 Tbsp. salt
½ cup shelled walnuts
2 cloves garlic
1 tsp. coriander seed
½ tsp. oregano, crushed
3 slices bread soaked in water
¼ cup water

Put in blender and whip until fine.
This sauce is added to various food preparations in small quantities. It is kept in a jar on the shelf in every Abkhasian kitchen to be used when necessary. It is also used as a condiment.

Walnut Sauce
½ lb. shelled walnuts (crushed in blender)
1 small onion cut in half

1 clove garlic
1 Tbsp. purpuljiga
4 slices bread (soaked in water)

Mix together in a bowl. Add water to thin just enough to be properly whipped in blender. Put in blender and whip in quantities according to the size of the blender until no lump is left in it. You will obtain a sauce with the consistency of an ordinary porridge.

Plum Sauce
1 lb. unripened green plums (Boil in one cup water until cooked. Let cool; clean out all the seeds.)
1 cup fresh sweet yogurt
½ tsp. purpuljiga
2 green onions (chopped fine)
1 Tbsp. green coriander (Chinese parsley)

Stir until mixed.

Yogurt Sauce
1 cup yogurt
½ tsp. purpuljiga

Stir until mixed.

ABUSTAH (mush)
This is a thick heavy meal obtained from boiling and kneading, with a wooden spoon, a coarsely ground cereal. It is commonly made from corn, millet or wheat, and is eaten as a side dish, like bread is eaten.

Corn Abustah
Bring to boil 5 cups of water. Turn down to medium heat. Add corn flour while stirring with wooden spoon. Keep adding flour slowly until it becomes the consistency of bread dough. Keep

stirring and turning over and over in the cooker for five to ten minutes until cooked.

Millet Abustah
Same as above, using whole millet.

Wheat Abustah
Bring to boil 5 cups of water. Add 1 cup fine cracked bulgur. When it comes up again to boiling, put the heat down to medium low. Leave it there for 20 minutes until the water is absorbed by the wheat. Stir with a wooden spoon for 10 minutes until cooked.

MEAT

Sun-dried Meat
Pieces of meat of various sizes, commonly 1" to 2" thick, 5" to 8" wide, 1' to 3' long are covered with a thin layer of purpuljiga and hung in the sunshine for a week or two. They are taken in at night.

Dried meat can be preserved for a long time when kept cool.

To serve, carve into small shavings, pour on walnut sauce and serve cool.

It is also eaten dipped in plum or yogurt sauce.

Smoked Meat
In winter time, when sun-drying is not possible, the same process is done by hanging meat pieces in the fireplace, which is built very high in Abkhasian style. It is served the same way.

Raw Meatballs
1 lb. minced meat (without fat)
½ lb. cracked wheat (soaked in water for one night)
2 tsp. purpuljiga

Mix and knead for 15 minutes. Shape into reasonably sized balls. Let rest for half an hour. Serve cool to be eaten dipped in plum or yogurt sauce.

Cooked Meat
Meat in pieces or minced meat in balls is cooked either by broiling or steaming and served warm with abustah and plum sauce or yogurt sauce.

Fish
All kinds of food preparation done with meat can also be done with fish.

Chicken
All kinds of food preparation done with meat can also be done with chicken. But I will describe here one particular dish which is considered a national Abkhasian dish and is known and appreciated in most parts of the Old World under the name of Abkhasian Chicken.

Abkhasian Chicken
Boil one chicken until cooked. De-bone it and break the meat into bite-sized pieces. Sauté it in a little butter with 1 medium sized onion (chopped fine). Dilute ½ lb. walnut sauce with chicken broth down to thickness of a thick soup. Pour the sauce on chicken in the cooker. Stir once. Leave on medium heat just to start bubbling. Take it off to the serving bowl. Let it cool and serve.

VEGETABLES
Most of the vegetables which are eaten raw are eaten raw in the form of a salad. The vegetables are made physically eatable by grating or cutting into small pieces. They then are garnished with one of the sauces according to taste and are served together with any kind of abustah.

Beans are boiled in water, and then mashed and mixed with walnut sauce.

PASTRY
Haluva

a) mix together
1 lb. minced beef
1 medium sized onion, grated
salt and black pepper to taste
½ cup water

b) make soft dough, adding water as necessary and knead
5 cups all-purpose flour
2 tsp. salt
1 egg
Let both rest for 1 hour.

Divide the dough into two; flatten each piece with a rolling pin to 1½" thick sheet. Cut the sheet into 2½" square pieces. Put on the middle of each piece 1 tsp. of the mixture (a), fold the layer over it, seal the ends by pressing with your fingers all around. Do the same to the other half of the dough.
Boil water in a large cooker (half filled). Put 1 Tbsp. salt into it.
Place the above prepared triangles into the boiling water—carefully and separately, none sticking to the other. Boil until cooked. When cooked, the pieces come to the surface.
Take them out with a filter scoop. Put them in a wide bowl; pour on enough yogurt sauce to cover. Melt butter in a pot with 1 tsp. paprika, scatter it over the dish. Serve warm.

DESSERT
Pumpkin in Oven

Peel the pumpkin. Slice it into 5" to 6" long and ½" thick pieces. Lay them in a pan in two layers. Pour on honey to your taste. Put 3 Tbsp. butter in small pieces on the pumpkin. Put it in the oven at 375 degrees. Bake until cooked. Leave it to cool down to room temperature. Sprinkle crushed walnuts on it and serve.

Chapter Two
PSYCHOLOGICAL MAN

In this chapter we shall be dealing with mind in its manifestation in three levels of subtlety: intellectual, spiritual and psychic.

As it is necessary to purify the physical system of physical refuse to enable man to cope successfully with the task of living his physical life, so it is also necessary to purify the psychological system from psychological refuse to enable man to cope successfully with the task of living his relationship with his environment and to overcome triumphantly his problems related to his vocational, familial, parental, conjugal, social and personal activities.

The psychological refuse of man appears in many forms such as anger, jealousy, doubt, meanness, hate, vindictiveness, selfishness, injustice, cruelty, arrogance, impatience, and fear of loss. There is only one single purifier for all of these forms of psychological refuse, and it is unconditional love.

Now, all the problems lie in how to reach this unconditional love. First of all, what is love?

Love is a cosmic field, electro-magnetic in nature, in which we live, function and express ourselves. Love manifests itself in the human being in three forms: eros love, philos love, and agape love.

EROS LOVE

This is love for the lovable. Anything which resonates with our sense of beauty and pleasure is lovable, like a beautiful flower pleasing the sense of smell with its fragrance and pleasing the sense of vision with its external beauty.

PHILOS LOVE

This is love engendered by a mutual interest. Two people having fondness for and attraction and involvement with the same thing such as, let us say, hockey, music, poetry, religion, or philosophy, will be attracted to each other because they find an opportunity for sharing the same thing together. The stronger and deeper the sharing, the more intense shall be the attraction. Man never feels complete by himself; no matter how much he enjoys experiencing something, he will comprehend one half of its expression and he will look for another person as his other half to make the expression complete. This is one fundamental law of love: *sharing*.

AGAPE LOVE

This is the kind of love which is engendered by belonging to, being one with, and our awareness of being one with something. The best and living example of this is the love of a mother for her child. The case of the awareness of the mother, that the child belongs to her and she belongs to it, is undoubtedly a reality. They are part of one another. This is unconditional love; this is a reflection of self-love. The notion of "you and me" totally disappears in its powerful warmth. All the psychological refuse disappears and melts in it. The child of a mother may be the ugliest creature in the world, but the mother will still love it; unconditionally. If we can attain the absolute awareness of our oneness with the whole creation, of our being an integral part of creation, and link ourselves with the Eternal Spirit of Creative Power, we can attain the power of Agape Love for everything existing in nature. Duality disappears, no "you and me" is left, everything becomes one, everything stems out from the same Eternal Spirit of Creative Power. An unprecedented awareness of brotherhood takes place and prevails spontaneously in all facets of our lives. We have no more psychological shit. We come to the point of loving even our enemy, as Jesus said. We reach the at-one-ment with the Maker and the Made that we are part of, and *egotism disappears*. Egotism is the psychological toxin, the mother of all darkness, negativity, failure, sickness and sin in Man.

To reach this stage of awareness requires education, edification, training and the experience of years under right coaching. It is a process of submission to a mature person in whom the student recognizes Higher Self manifesting and through whom the student learns to submit his lower self to the Higher Self. It may appear to be obedience to another person, but it is actually submission to one's own Self. Anyone wanting to know more about this subject should read the chapter entitled "Sufism" in my book *I Come From Behind Kaf Mountain* (also published by Threshold Books).

For readers who have further quests, I will keep myself freely open to their questions. Freely I received, freely I shall give; aspiration is yours and it is costly; the price of it is your Ego.

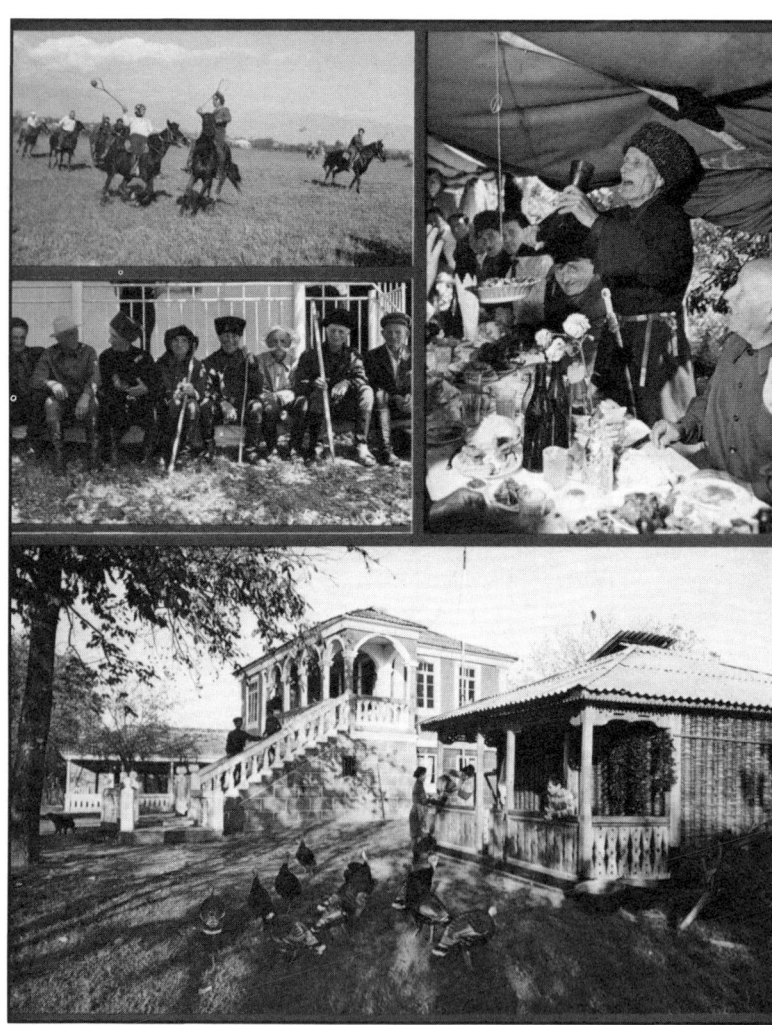

Chapter Three
ECOLOGICAL MAN

The purpose of keeping man functioning in his entirety—healthily, vigorously, fittingly and harmoniously—is to enable man to better cope in his relationships with his environment.

All the rules in the discipline of longevity and well-being may be observed and, as a result, a long-living, vigorous, healthy and harmonious human being is raised. But unless this individual achieves triumphant results in daily life in his environment, all the effort and energy spent will be for naught. He will be like a carburetor manufactured by a factory to be of the highest individual qualities, but not put in the system of the machinery of a car. What will be the value of this high-quality product if it is only to stay on the shelf of the warehouse?

A well-fit man will reach an abundant life, and reaching an abundant life will further encourage and motivate this man to keep fit; let us not forget, a tree without fruit shall be burnt in the fireplace, and such a man will be better off in the grave.

I shall tackle one by one some of the main ecological aspects of human life.

THE PHYSICAL ASPECT
OF HUMAN ECOLOGY

The physical aspect of the ecology of man consists of dealing with nature, the resistance of the body to external effects such as cold, heat, germs and pollution which naturally and inevitably are around us in our daily life, and endurance of the body to the physical activities we have to get involved with to conduct our natural daily chores in order to exist. We have to condition, train and help our bodies to victoriously confront these inevitably present adverse elements in our environment. The idea is not to keep our system toxin-free, germ-free, and pollution-free by staying away from these things, but it is rather to enable our bodies to handle them and make them harmless in proper ways.

THE VOCATIONAL ASPECT OF HUMAN ECOLOGY

Our vocational success is closely related to our keeping a toxin-free system, since a toxin-free nervous system functions as a better home and reflector of our mind. A very noticeable increase of intelligence is experienced after purification from toxins in the system. Our intellectual mind starts functioning better, our reasoning ability increases, and the way is opened to the subconscious mind, to which our spiritual and psychic faculties belong. Elimination of psychological toxin becomes more possible and, as a result, a more loving, tolerant, congenial personality takes shape, enabling a positive and productive cooperation in teamwork and getting along better with co-workers.

THE SOCIAL ASPECT OF HUMAN ECOLOGY

All our social involvements are in general overlapped with our vocational life. Most of the human relationships we build up come from our business activities: office parties, dinners, luncheons, picnics, private visits, etc. In most vocations, expanding our business, building up clientele, and finding new leads for new business are very much dependent on how active and harmonious we keep ourselves in our social life. An introverted person who leads a solitary and privacy-oriented life is very likely to make a poor individual for success of all kinds. Man is a gregarious being; sharing and being popular enriches human life. To be able to perpetuate such a life, one has to be a congenial, loving, altruistic, harmonious person, totally and absolutely free from all kinds of psychological toxins. To be able to keep a trouble-free and discrepancy-free human relationship, one has to know how to give, forgive and love. Love is the key word.

THE FAMILIAL ASPECT OF HUMAN ECOLOGY

Family is the backbone of Abkhasian life. The most eloquent meaning of the saying "one for all, and all for one" reflects itself in Abkhasian family life. Abkhasian mentality is not an individualistic one, but rather it is a strongly communalistic one. I would like to make this notion very clear; its being understood accurately is important. The value of the individual is very important. Abkhasian culture produced strong and highly endowed individuals throughout all its history, but the crucible of the individual value is communal sharing, in all kinds of groups, starting from the smallest—the family—to village, country, nation and eventually to mankind and the universe.

In the family, every member has his place and role distinctly determined, and is given responsiblity and credit for that. He knows that he has a function; he is doing something useful which contributes to the family and he is needed. This state of being keeps him active and efficient. When a true Abkhasian encounters making a choice between his individual good and the family good, he will unshakably choose the latter.

Two North American scientists, Dr. Sula Benet and Alexander Leaf, M.D., who visited Abkhasia to conduct research on the longevity of its people, were both much impressed by the Abkhasian family system. They came close to believing that the main reason for the longevity of these people was that elderly people held the concrete belief of being needed so strongly that this conviction linked them to life. Dr. Sula Benet wrote two books on the subject: *How to Live to Be 100*, The Dial Press 1976, New York, and *Abkhasians, The Long-Living People of the Caucasus*, Holt, Rinehart and Winston, New York. Dr. Alexander Leaf wrote an article in the January, 1973 issue of *National Geographic*. Should the reader wish more detailed accounts, I would recommend these publications.

THE PARENTAL ASPECT OF HUMAN ECOLOGY

One of the most important factors in the structure of family life is the harmonious relationship between parents and children. The homogeneity of tradition, mentality and behavior in a society contributes tremendously to a well-maintained relationship in the family, especially between parents and children. This condition is difficult to obtain in North American communities. The values in one family usually differ to a great extent from those in other families of the community because of the differences in each family's background. The stage of being a homogeneous nation is not reached yet, and reaching this stage seems to be a slow process. Whatever the values taught at home, they do not link up with those observed outside the family, at school, on the street, on the playgrounds and so on. What we call nowadays the "generation gap" is more a "social gap," because out there in the society, whatever prevails is nothing but confusion. If in here, at home, there is a certain well established system, it will certainly be different from what is out there, and the child will stray in between. There will be a natural gap between clarity and confusion. Since being confused is normally easier than being clear, the child gets confused, and we call it a generation gap.

Under these conditions, divergence between parent and child develops into such a heart-breaking thing that all kinds of sicknesses, troubles and life-long suffering take place. All these problems are very well known to all of us here in the West.

The character of the parent-child relationship in Abkhasian tradition is totally beyond application here in the West. To go into detail on it will not have any practical purpose. Having any problem in the parent-child relationship in an Abkhasian community is unheard of, but if the Abkhasian system were applied to North America, it would cause nothing but trouble. This is a social problem and will not be solved by the determination of one single individual. But, to give an idea, I will explain it in short.

The genuine mutual respect and love which prevail in a traditional Abkhasian family can be duplicated nowhere in the world. The authority of the father is unshakable. The father is not allowed to show an open and manifest expression of love to the child, but deep down in the atmosphere of home, there is nothing but a vibration of love and recognition and respect for one another, backed up by this love, which itself seems invisible. The social relationship between father and son, and mother and daughter, is a kind of master and apprentice relationship, and displays every aspect of this kind of relationship. Because there is no discrepancy between in-home teaching and the teaching which prevails outside the home in the society, whatever the growing child observes and learns about the facts of life at home is applicable out there in the society. The beauty, pleasure, satisfaction, peace of mind and happiness brought about by such a relationship reflects its effects on the health and well-being of the individuals. This one fact which contributes to longevity is unfortunately inapplicable in much more complex societies like the North American ones. So, in short, we had better forget about this aspect of Abkhasian life, and look at it as one watermelon in the field of the summer to come.

THE CONJUGAL ASPECT
OF HUMAN ECOLOGY

One important aspect of our life which has great effect on our health, happiness and longevity is the sexual aspect. It may look more proper to tackle this subject as an independent fact, not necessarily confined to our conjugal life. But considering the highest form of its manifestation and at the same time remaining faithful and respectful to the purpose of nature, namely perpetuation of species, I thought it proper to include it here.

When we come together as man and woman to share our life, we have many involvements to handle together which are as important as our sharing sex. But since the most important motive, starter, and stimulator of conjugal life comes from sexual attraction, it is only sensible to believe that this starting factor should remain alive, important and well-manifested throughout our married life. Abkhasians are not sexual gluttons, but they certainly are sexual gourmets. It is a noticeable characteristic in every Abkhasian. It is strongly believed that no markedly high attainment of any kind can be achieved by an individual who is not successful and satisfied in his sex life.

I am going to outline the Abkhasian sexual teaching briefly, as much as I can within the scope of this book.

In Abkhasian teaching, sex is neither a dirty thing, nor a dirty topic to speak about; on the contrary, it is a physiological and psychological need which has to be fulfilled as intelligently, properly and wholly as possible. If even a little child asks a question of an elderly person concerning sexual matters, he will never be rebuked. He will be answered in a proper way, patiently and compassionately, according to the degree of his grasp and without giving an evasive answer, as in any other physiological and psychological matter, using pertinent examples from the animal kingdom.

In sex edification, special emphasis is put on the distinctive differences between male and female sexuality. The well-recommended golden rule, "do unto others as you would like it to be done unto you," does not apply in sharing sex. We should not find ourselves feeding our horse with beefsteak because we ourselves like beefsteak; we should know what our horse likes. This is one of the governing principles in Abkhasian sex edification.

We should be taught about the sexual peculiarities of the opposite sex, so that we know how to behave in order to be speaking the sexual language of our partner. On the animal level, a male ordinarily wants to reach discharge of the tension and pressure of sexual stimulus as soon as possible; the next thing is to turn his back and sleep. A young man needs to be instructed and trained to be stimulation-oriented rather than relief-oriented, as naturally a man is, but he can learn to enjoy being in a stimulated state of being.

Of course, because conjugal life involves two human beings it is a two-way street. As the male has be to informed and trained concerning the sexual peculiarities of the opposite sex and has to observe carefully the facts and behave accordingly, so has the female. The physiological and psychological functioning of the male sexuality is totally different from the same in the female, although there are also some common and overlapping areas.

To enjoy and be successful in the phenomenon of orgasm a man needs energy, vigor, and strength, because to be able to do it he needs the necessary energy to produce an erection as well as energy to produce the chemical substance to ejaculate. Therefore, he should be in his best form when he is rested. Woman, on the other hand, needs to be relaxed. As a result, a woman will like having sex in the evening after a day's work, whereas a man will be more ready in the morning. To deal with this discrepancy, education, teaching, and training is needed.

And there are certain things that will turn a man off very easily, which will reduce even a young and vigorous man to an impotent situation. First of all, it is best if love-making is not too premeditated. It should come as the unavoidable course of action of a certain mutual vibration gaining momentum, rather than as a too aggressive proposal.

Special care should be taken to eliminate all kinds of inhibitions in sexual encounters. Any difficulty which may arise between partners should be openly and frankly shared with the earnestness of a positive attitude. Partners should shun making fun of each other. Gentleness, compassion, patience, aptness and tactfulness are especially the responsibility of the male. A woman is like a musical instrument with one thousand strings; a good musician should know how to strike each single one of them and get the proper tune. The man is taught about all of these things for his own benefit, for the sake of having pleasure for himself. Nothing should be practiced in sexual intercourse by man for the purpose of pleasing woman, but whatever he does to please himself should spontaneously please woman. If the woman senses that her partner is striving to please her, if he himself is not pleased, the intercourse will lose all its charm for her. For woman, the warmth of togetherness, caresses of all kinds, by hands, by words, by tongue, and by lips are as important and pleasing as orgasm; man should know this and behave accordingly. Considering the natural superficiality and shallowness of man in sexual manifestation, he needs a lot of edification to be able to cope with the nature-given depth of woman. Once he attains it, he shall meet his heaven.

Let us face it, all the consequences of one sexual intercourse of the shortest duration for a woman is nine months, whereas if a man can make sexual intercourse last nine minutes, he is a champion. What a comparison. Man can overcome his shallowness only by being edified and refined under proper coaching, and in Abkhasian tradition, it is thought well worthwhile. Had I to write everything on Abkhasian sexual teaching, it would make a book three to four hundred pages by itself; maybe one day I will do it. Here, for now, I just wanted to outline the general principles to show how much bearing it is believed to have on human well-being. It is very difficult to relate comprehensively the whole of the teaching without going into detailed and descriptive explanations, and without bringing about many examples from factual aspects of life.

* * *

So far I have only described sexuality in its regulatory aspect—in other words, as a function which helps human beings to regulate their physical and psychological well-being. When both members of a couple have reached the state of direct communion with God, another dimension of Man enters the field of existence. The sexual act, in the case of such a couple, becomes a cosmic act in which the partners are the points of contact of two halves uniting to form a whole. The marriage becomes *the marriage in heaven*. The orgasm experienced becomes a wholly comprehensive one. Partners are melted in it. They come out of it with an experience very similar to the case of a person waking up from a knock-out. It is not a sensation related to the genital system only but involving the whole nervous system from the toes to the top of the head. It is very physical in nature, but a seemingly invisible part of extreme subtlety vibrates and throbs and the partners feel like two joyful rivers running into each other. There is no duplicate for such an intercourse. It is like the gods having intercourse as it is depicted in ancient Greek mythology. Sex is fulfilled in its wholeness and it becomes a Divine experience. Such a couple is capable of living the ideal monogamic life purely, genuinely and naturally free of any trace of hypocrisy.

Now, in today's marriage laws in the West, this monogamy we expect from every married couple. We are expecting the impossible. The result is failure and frustration.

In establishing a harmonious and lasting togetherness, our observations should be based on realistic facts. If we base our expectations and evaluations on some idealistic, man-made rules, ignoring the mighty manifestations of natural laws, we are doing nothing but looking for a utopia and exposing ourselves to frustrating disappointments.

I am not trying to prove anything here; nor am I imposing something I believe on others. I am only relating what is the Abkhasian establishment of marriage and the governing basis behind it. Not even one case of divorce in any traditional Abkhasian community was ever heard of in their history. According to the statement made by Dr. Pitirim Sorokin, sociologist, Harvard University, in 1972: "Two of every five marriages in recent years in the U.S.A. end in divorce." And furthermore, in 1982, this percentage was declared as three of every five marriages, a 60% divorce rate; and it is increasing, let us keep this in mind. Abkhasian and North Americans are the same human beings; the only difference is that the former respect the natural laws, while the latter insist on some man-made laws, expecting from human beings something which is impossible from nature's point of view.

If we have a look at the animal kingdom to observe how male and female sexuality functions, we observe some very interesting facts. Even for the most vigorous of the species, the female copulates only once or twice a year, depending on the length of time of the gestation and nursing period. After having copulated, she completely stops her sexual activities and assumes the role of expecting and later nursing mother. The male goes around and inseminates other females. Both male and female, to fulfill their repective roles concerning their sexual life, are endowed with behaviors commensurate with these roles. As I expressed earlier, female sexual psychology is deeper, more substantial, more stable and conscientious, whereas the male's is more superficial, evasive, and noncommittal. Even in the case of wildlife where male and female live as couples sharing the responsiblity of the togetherness in some set-up similar to marriage, while the male keeps faithful to his committment to his home, he still keeps in touch with the casual adventures of the outside life, with its touch of sexuality.

Whether animal or human, male and female sexuality have separate characteristics similar to what is described above. Considering these as unchangeable and inescapable laws of nature, various human societies tried to establish an institution of marriage practicable enough, considering nature's dictate and, at the same time, able to bring some fair order to social functions.

In the earlier times of human social life, conjugal life was polygamous in favor of man. Social and religious rules were established supporting polygamy, trying to make it work in justice, righteousness and fairness. Christian law was polygamic, suggesting only that the clergymen should be monogamous. General acceptance of monogamous marriage in the Western world did not come as a rule of Christianity, but rather as a result of the manifesto of human rights, which later on took shape under what is called the Napoleonic Code and then the Civil Code. Monogamous marriage developed and got established as a generally accepted system during the last three to four hundred years in the Christian world, not without creating a lot of tragic, catastrophic and sad results at times. In cases where monogamy seemed to be working quite well, it brought in a lot of hypocrisy to conjugal life. This is nothing but adultery within marriage. According to the Abkhasian judgment of values, adultery is defined as the lack of equality in sexual relations. It is considered an adultery when one marriage partner consents to enter sexual intercourse just to please the other. It is adultery when one person uses another just to relieve themselves. Any sexual relationship that produces guilt in at least one of the parties is also adulterous. It is not the fact that a relationship outside of marriage takes place, but the fact that one person is not emancipated enough to be involved without guilt.

* * *

One of the greatest killers of success, harmony and happiness in conjugal life is the power of jealousy and possessiveness which develops as a result of seemingly well-attained sexual fitness. When a young man is well edified and trained as an ideal sexual partner for a woman, the woman who lives her sexual experience with such a man gets attached to him as a unique meaning of her life. When woman, who is fastidious by nature in her sexuality, meets a perfect mate, she develops such an attachment to him that she strongly tends to be jealous and possessive to the extent of making an elephant out of every flea. She sticks like a Siamese twin to the man, unwilling even to recognize the most legitimate space to him. Such a woman will be incorrigible if given any chance to develop further in her demands. Man will feel suffocated from lack of space. It becomes a very difficult, if not impossible, case to handle. Only a unanimous and uniform social attitude towards such a situation will save the marriage. No matter how much mutual love prevails between couples, such jealousy and possessiveness will not stop separation; it will make it worse. As the English writer W. Somerset Maugham puts it in his book *The Razor's Edge*: "When a woman falls in love, she ceases to be lovable."

In the Abkhasian tradition, the institution of marriage is established giving full consideration to the natural phenomena which are inevitable anyway. Contrary to the rest of the known world, throughout history polygamy was never accepted and practiced in Abkhasian tradition. The Abkhasian woman would never share her husband with another wife. She is the only boss of her home. She expects faithfulness from her husband to his commitments and responsibilities to the home she is sharing with him. Outside of home, she recognizes unlimited space and freedom to him. His getting involved with other women does not bother her at all. She does not question her husband; she does not spy on him. His flirting, joking, having intimacy with other women in the society makes her proud. Even in the presence of his wife, he openly flirts with the surrounding ladies. His wife knows confidently that whatever happens with other women is a transient affair, never affecting her conjugal life. If an Abkhasian man neglects his wife and gives his preference to another woman, it is an unfortunate weakness and shame for him; but she shows compassion and understanding. Such a situation is extremely rare.

On the other hand, the wife also enjoys great freedom. As long as she keeps her name respectable in the society, she is considered a decent person. No woman who can handle her life intelligently will be insulted.

No woman likes to be seen and known as a jealous and possessive wife. This is a sign of weakness and trespassing the rights of another human being. It is believed that nobody can own another human being no matter what their relationship—husband, wife, child, parent, friend, or whatever. Because your Maker does not possess you, does not interfere in your free choice, how can any human being possess another?

There is no reason to be jealous in matters concerning love if what one is experiencing is real love. Love is infinite, therefore indivisible. By loving many people instead of loving one, one is not giving love to any one of them by taking away some of the love from the other. If one loves one, one gives all one's love to this one; then if one loves another, one gives all one's love to this one also, without

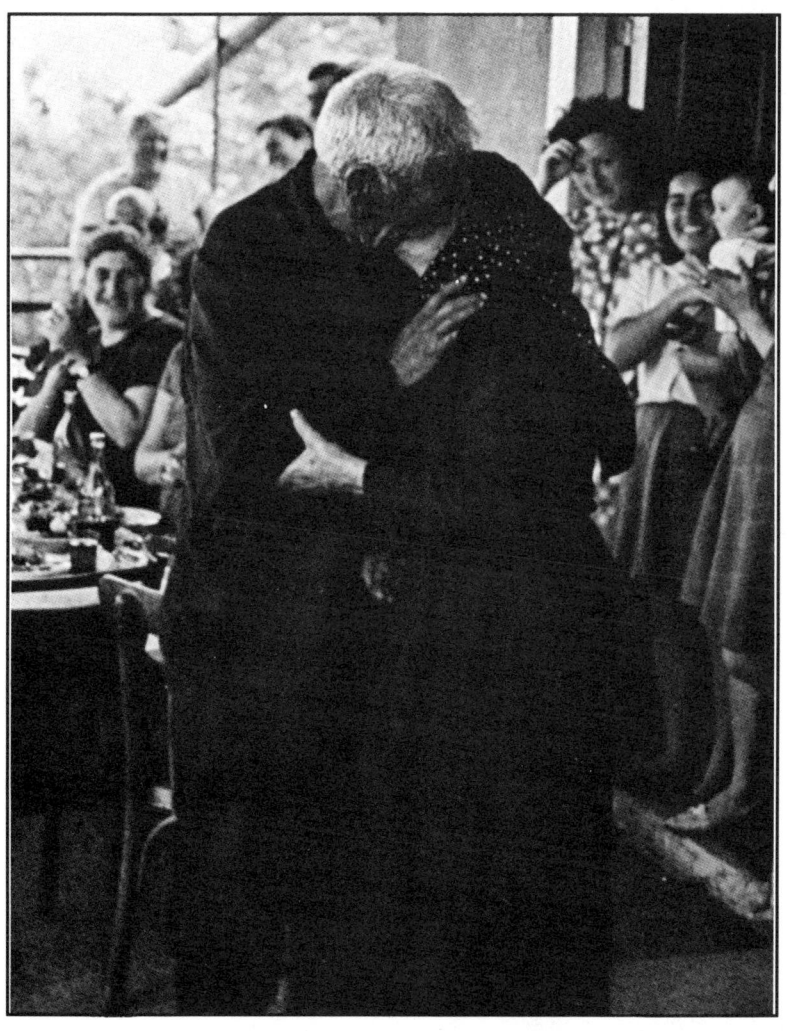
Karum, 95, hugs his wife Keke, 80.

taking anything from the other. Because love is infinite it is therefore indivisible. By definition, infinity divided by ten is equal to infinity divided by a million.

In practical life, we experience this state with our children. If we have ten children, we give all our love to each one of them; we do not divide our love into ten smaller portions and give one tenth to each child. We may not like them equally, but we love them equally. We should not confuse liking and loving.

Understanding and agreeing with this concept of love is not easy; it depends on the definition of love we have and we were given starting from our early childhood. For the last twenty-one years I have lived as a North American and I know that it will be difficult if not impossible for a North American to be pliant to the concept. But also, I am an Abkhasian, and I know that it works for Abkhasians. I am not in a position to favor one or the other for anybody. Each one has to be his own judge and make his own decisions. The fact is that the Abkhasian concept of love brings harmony and endurance to an Abkhasian marriage, and takes away a lot of what we call psychological toxins from our system, whereas 60% of North American marriages end in divorce.

Try to get the truth, if you want to understand Abkhasian longevity. You are eligible for it also, if you can get it.

THE PERSONAL ASPECT OF HUMAN ECOLOGY

What I mean by the Personal aspect of our ecological function is the ability of our personality to fit our ecological conditions. As human beings, we have two states of being, with which we *are*: our Essence and our Personality. Some of the manifestations we display come from our Essence and some come from our Personality. It is very important to make clear what is our Essence and what is our Personality. Our Essence is what we have vested, stored, treasured in us, as utilizably good. Our Personality is our state in which we developed and made manifest our Essence. In

Ecological Man

other words, our Personality is our Essence activated to meet our ecology. Essence is inherited, Personality is made from it. Essence is latent; Personality is active. Let me give a practical example. Let us take the case of a race horse. A race horse has the essence vested in it to be a race horse, but to develop the Personality of a race horse, it has to be trained, conditioned, exercised and raised to be successful in action on the race track. If the Essence is not developed, it may still manifest itself at random, occasionally and incidentally, but it will always be whimsical. When a Personality is developed from the Essence with proper and right coaching, the chances for victory will be increased.

A human being with a Personality well developed to meet his ecology, which actually is the task of living, shall live an abundant and long life in full potency.

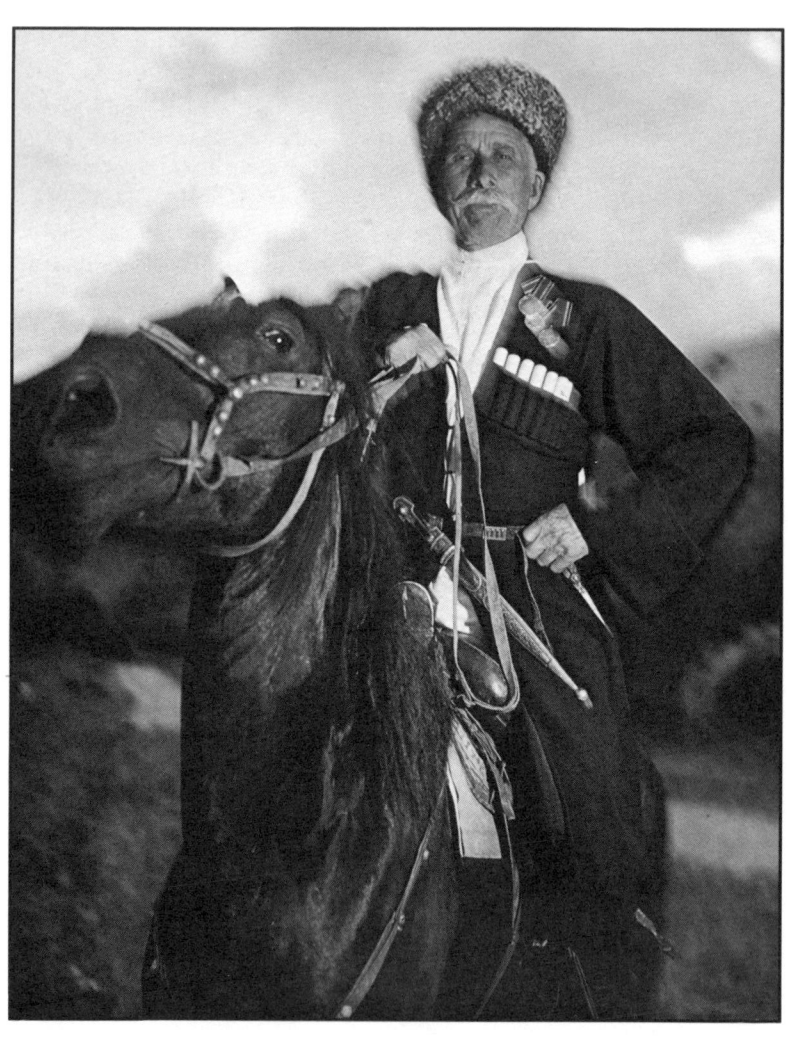

One of Abkhasia's many spirited centenarians.

EVERYTHING HAS ITS PLACE

Abkhasians believe and preach that whatever you do, you concentrate yourself on this one thing and you do it properly. They also teach that everything has its place. There is nothing good or bad as it is. Everything is evaluated according to its appropriateness. For example, in some instances when you kill, you become a murderer; in other instances when you kill, you become a hero. Is killing good or bad? Always the answer will be: "It depends." When you are in the family as a woman of responsibility of the house—in other words, when you are the lady of the house—you have to be ladylike. When you are with your man (for we don't have a word for husband in our language—we say, "my man" or "my woman"), you have to be as good a bitch as possible. You have to be bitchy; ladylike behavior doesn't fit when you are with your man. So everything has its place, and there's a reason for that.

There is an Abkhasian epic about a warrior named the Dev-yapsh. In the old days, according to custom, when there was going to be a collective campaign, various chieftains would come with their entourage to another chieftain's castle, and they would say, "We are going to do this and this, or hit such and such a country. Will you join us?" And then if the chieftain wanted to, he would join, and the chieftains and their entourage would continue like this until they would grow like an avalanche, and then they would go to hit that place.

Various chieftains came with their entourage to call on this warrior for a collective campaign. They came to him because he was known as a very good warrior and they wanted to have him. His castle was located high on a mountain, and down in front of it there was a beautiful plain. The chieftains and their entourage camped there, and they sent two men up to the castle to find the Dev-yapsh to invite him to join the campaign.

The two men went up and found the Dev-yapsh in a small pool, giving a bath to his woman.

"Oh," they said, "we came at the wrong time." And they slowly went away.

They waited, and when they came back a little bit later, they found the Dev-yapsh sitting with his woman in an antechamber next to the bathroom. He was braiding her hair; combing and braiding, and playing with her and giving her some attention.

The men said, "We came at the wrong time," and they went away again. And they wondered, "How will this special man—this warrior— fight?"

And then they came a third time, and found the Dev-yapsh sitting and eating grapes and pears in a very comfortable way, and his woman was playing the lute and singing for him.

The men went out and from outside they shouted, "Hey, anybody at home? Anybody at home?" They were thinking that there would be no entry. They were fed up with waiting.

The Dev-yapsh came out and said, "What can I do for you?"

The men gave the message: "Such and such a king, such and such a king, and such and such a king are here organizing a collective raid, and would like you to join them."

And the Dev-yapsh said, "I'm coming."

When the two men descended from the mountain on their horses and came out onto the plain, they saw that the Dev-yapsh was already there. They said, "Hey, how has this man who is so fond of his wife detached himself so quickly? He even came before us! How did he arrange his saddle, his saddlebag, his powder supply and bullet supply and everything he needs to be so prepared?" They were amazed.

"Where are your men?" they asked. He had one horse and himself.

"I have no men. I fight single."

And so the chieftains and their entourage fought the campaign, engaging in many battles and meeting with difficulties. The whole raid was a success because of the strategic and heroic accomplishments of the Dev-yapsh. The chieftains eventually returned to the

Ecological Man   53

plain below the Dev-yapsh's castle. The Dev-yapsh said, "I would like to invite you to stay with me for a few days."

The chieftains said, "We had better continue on our way, but we should have a one-day stay here to do our accounting," as was customary. They pitched their camp, and then they said, "Look, if it wasn't for you, this battle wouldn't be won. So we are making you the toastmaster and the judge of the meeting. Everything actually belongs to you. You make the distribution; if you give us something, all right."

The Dev-yapsh agreed, and he said, "Where are those two men you sent to call me in the first place?" The two men came. "These two men know me better than the rest of you. Whatever they feel is appropriate for me to be given, I want these two men to give me."

The chieftains had attacked a Russian headquarters and they had also captured many human beings as war prisoners to be sold in the slave bazaars in Damascus, as was the custom. Among the prisoners was the daughter of the Russian general. The two men said, "This is one thing you would be very fond of, so we give you this girl."

"All right," the Dev-yapsh said, and took the girl. "All the rest of the things are yours, because I got the most precious thing. These two men would tell you why." He took the girl on his horse, and went to his home.

Two seasons later the Russian general, knowing the story of the Caucasians, sent word to the chieftain who had organized the raid. No matter what happened, or how many leaders joined a campaign, the campaign still went on the name of the organizing chieftain who started it. The Russian general sent word that he was coming to ransom his daughter; he wanted her kept so that she wouldn't be sold somewhere.

Two seasons after that the general came to the chieftain, and he was told that his daughter had been left with the Dev-yapsh. The chieftain received the general as his guest because the general came with the necessary goods to pay for and rescue his daughter. Now that they were friends, the chieftain accompanied the general to the

Dev-yapsh's place. And when they came to the Dev-yapsh's place, they asked for the girl. The Dev-yapsh received them as his guests and called the girl. The girl came, and greeted her father. When her father told her of his intention, she said, "I'm not going away from here. I will stay here. I will become one of these people. I have never experienced the feeling of being at home and the feeling of being a respected woman anywhere else as much as I have felt here."

"Are you in love with the Dev-yapsh?" her father asked.

She said, "I am in love with him, but not as his woman."

Then the Dev-yapsh asked permission to talk, and he said, "Where are the two men they sent to me in the first place?"

The two men came, and the Dev-yapsh took them to his side and said, "Whatever I am going to tell you, these two men will be my witnesses. And in some things I am going to tell you, all of you will be my witnesses."

He said, "When I am in my home and with my woman I behave the way these two men will testify. When I am in the battlefield, when I am called to a fellowship, I will respond the way these two men and also the rest of you have witnessed. When I am in the battlefield, I fight the way you saw. And when I have a woman under my roof, I treat her as such. I don't confuse this woman with my wife."

So this is all I am saying. It ends this way. Everything has its place, at the right place, at the right time.

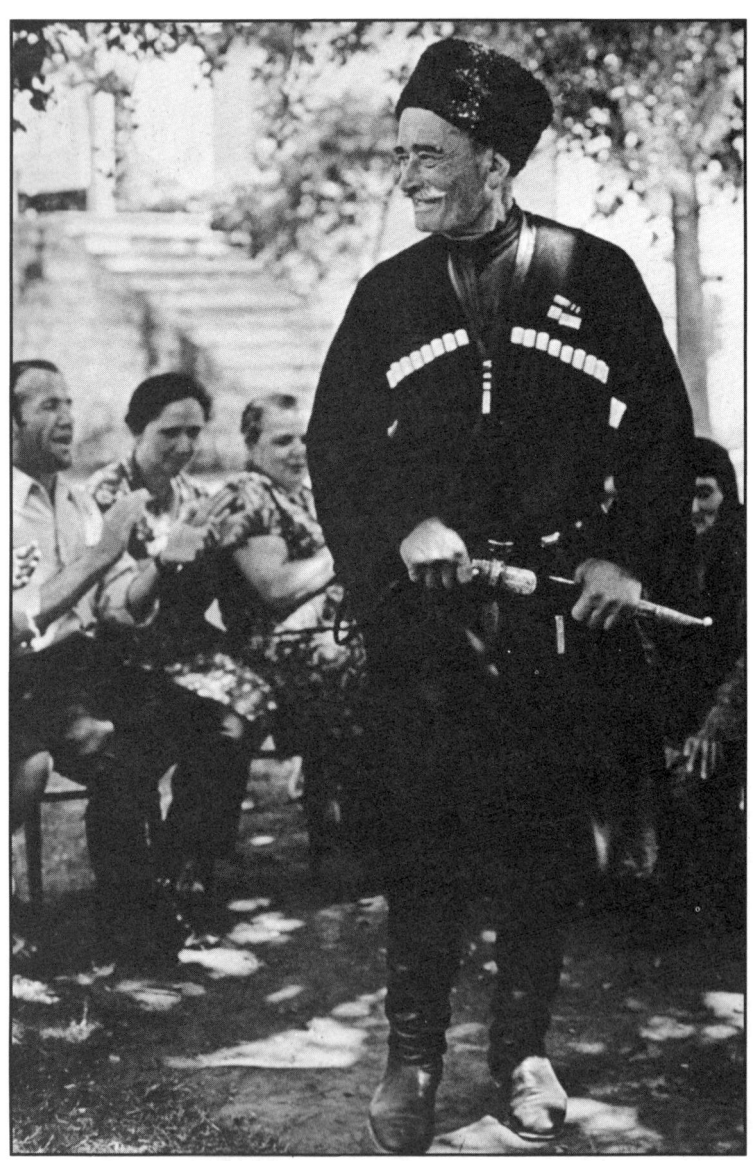

This gentleman is over 100 years old.

Chapter Four
MAN AS A WHOLE

In this chapter I shall give a brief account of the spiritual teaching of the Caucasus Mountains in its version as applied by Abkhasian people, who are one group among others, and by whom the mystical aspect of Man has been cultivated for thousands and thousands of years.

The precise meaning of "mystical" here is to be understood as a faculty peculiar to Man relating to or resulting from his direct communion with God or ultimate reality, which is neither apparent to the senses nor obvious to the intelligence, but which can be experienced through developing the finest receptivity down in the deepest realm of the subconscious mind. First, I would like to give the definitions of some key words frequently used in the teaching.

GOD

God is the unknowable ultimate reality which stands at the final, original end of every existing thing, object, matter and concept, and from which everything stems out, emanates and comes to life. In other words, the cause of life is called God. Just as simple as that. Instead of using a long phrase such as "the Cause of Life," we coined a word for it, and this word is "God." When we trace down to the origin of any given thing, to find how it started, we end up in God.

Let us take a simple example as an exercise. Suppose that the given thing is *me*. We ask the question: "Who made me?" and suppose that we answer this question as "my mother," because the only tangible, concrete, material thing we know is that I came out from my mother. This, everybody has seen; this cannot be denied or unseen and there is nothing mysterious about it. It is a sure thing, that I came out from my mother. So the answer is: "My mother made me."

Now the next question will be: "Who made my mother?" The answer is: "Her mother made her."

The next question comes as: "Who made her mother?" The answer: "Her mother."

If we continue asking the questions in the same manner, for one thousand years, still we will have the same answer. Depending on our patience, perseverance and endurance, at some point we shall be tired and say: "*I don't know.*" That very thing that you call "*I don't know,*" the Abkhasian wiseman calls God, the original *source of life*. Here, I would like to invite the reader to pay particular attention to what is said. By saying: "I don't know," we implicitly accept that there is something there, but we do not know it. By this, it becomes obvious that we don't deny God. We don't say there is nothing. We say there is something, but this thing we don't know. Now it becomes clear that our task is not to believe or not to believe in God: we already know that there is a God, but we don't *know* God.

So our task is not to believe in God, our task is to *know* God. To say "I believe in God" is as absurd as to say "I believe in mathematics." There is no such thing as believing in mathematics. You either know or don't know mathematics. The Abkhasian wiseman does not preach believing in God. He does not say to believe in God; he says: "Let us find God, the eternal and ultimate spirit of engendering or creative power."

The only way to find God is through mystical experience—mystical meaning the thing defined above. Please refer to it and read it once more slowly until it becomes clear to you and you thoroughly grasp it.

MAN

Man is the highest form, the masterpiece, the all-expressing product of this "eternal and ultimate spirit of creative power," or, for short, God.

Man as a Whole

Every life-bearing thing carries within it this life-giving force, and is conscious of it to the extent of the degree of awareness it is able to exercise. And this awareness manifests its highest degree in man, and the degree of this awareness can be cultivated to increase through certain spiritual exercises, education and edification. This is a science which has a discipline peculiar to itself. In Abhkasian language this science is called Ahmusta Kebzeh, "the discipline of the elect." Ahmusta Kebzeh is defined as a process of awakening and developing the latent faculties in man under Divine grace and guidance. It is a totally different teaching from the rest of the spiritual teachings of the world. Ahmusta Kebzeh is totally practical, scientific, mundane and down to earth. Its purpose is to train Man to live his life in full abundance and enjoy all his faculties in full application to better himself in every single avenue, field, and space of life. It looks fine, does it not, but it is the training and teaching of a lifetime and cannot be taught in books. Ahmusta Kebzeh is a work of processing, like swimming, bicycle riding, or musical instrument playing, which can be learned by doing, not just by studying. It cannot be my intention to teach here the spiritual message of the Mountains of the Caucasus, the home country of human myth, legend and wisdom; the home country of Greek mythology, of Zeus, of Mars, of Prometheus, of the Golden Fleece; the home country of the key to human secrets of creation and of its mysteries; the home country of Melchisedech who brought the divine message to Patriarch Abraham; the home country of the secrets of the Flood of Noah described in its twenty-six-thousand-year-old folk songs. No, I am not trying to do that in this little book. That is a thing which cannot be done in even one thousand books, anyhow.

But I shall give some fragments of it to cover the peculiarity of Holistic Man, without which the Abkhasian longevity would look like a broken glass. As I said in the beginning, we cannot take one human function out of five functions and by improving only that function bring the human being into wholeness and secure longevity and well-being.

When a man receives the training of this discipline, grasps it and graduates, making passing marks in every aspect of it, he becomes a *whole man*, a man using all his faculties, a completed man, a man who has reached a direct communion with God. So when we use the word "God," hear it always according to the definition and description of it given here. Forget about whatever is your concept of it according to your Sunday, Saturday or Friday School teaching. Forget or unlearn this concept temporarily in order to apply yourself to the task of following what I am saying.

Now, because everything existing in the universe is emanated from God, God is everywhere and in everything. Without God being in it, nothing can exist and have life.

As I said, our task was finding God. If we are looking for something which can be found everywhere, we would look for it in the place which is closest to us. If God is everywhere, omnipresent, It is also in us; so instead of looking for God in the sky, we would be better off looking in ourselves, and apparently we would have a better chance to reach God. Now, do we have the necessary ability to do this job? Ahmusta Kebzeh says that we have, but it is latent, dormant, and we have to awaken and develop it. When it is done, we are one with God. We are one with God anyhow, just because we live; but what we miss is our tangible awareness of our oneness. It is this awareness that we strive to reach. Our body becomes a vehicle for God whether we know it or not, but our knowing it, and having a tangible awareness of it, makes all the difference.

This life-giving force which is in us we call soul. Ahmusta Kebzeh says this soul is the thing we talk about when we say "I" or "I am." Ahmusta Kebzeh teaches us to say: "I am a Soul and I have a body." Not that I am a body and I have a soul. This is one point which needs to be grasped solidly:

"*I am a soul and I have a body.*"

The body is the vehicle of the soul which is me. In Biblical language, "the body is the temple of God." So actually, if we have attained the *truth*, if we really know in full awareness what we are talking about, when we say "I" we are saying "God." But let us be careful. This is not for everybody; this is only for those who are *aware*, and not intellectually aware, but inwardly aware.

Now, I want to come back to the effect of spiritual development in practical life.

Cosmic *mind* individualized and incarnated in Man develops in two opposite, up and down, directions. These two aspects of Mind are respectively called Spiritualized Mind and Materialized Mind. These two developments can also be called respectively, Godization leading to Union with the Essence, and Satanization leading to separation from the Essence. The Human Being who is in the process of Godization comes to the realization of One God; the Human Being who is in the process of Satanization comes to the realization of two gods, the second one being himself, singled out, separate. When this is the case, the first God gradually fades away and the person becomes Satan-possessed.

The Human Being who is in the process of Godization becomes one with the Cosmos, which contains the Essence and all witnesses in a collective existence or at-one-ment. He journeys toward Oneness and develops the "I" within. He is led by Love into contact with his fellow-man and with all witnesses. The man who is in the process of Satanization only develops his *ego*.

There are two directions in which the human Mind may develop. This represents a vertical scale of subtlety. The tendency of flow is from higher to lower according to Cosmic gravity. Our attraction is most naturally toward coarser planes, which is to say, to earthly existence, unless we experience some uplifting agency. In light of this short explanation, it can easily be seen that the human Mind tends toward materialization, and this, as a result, brings about the development of *Ego* rather than *I*.

The egotistical Man will preserve his gregarious or communally oriented tendency as long as it fits his individual profit and benefit. Therefore primitive people had to stick together to survive adverse conditions of all sorts. They willingly shared life in its wholeness because they were under the force of circumstances.

They were fully aware of the tangible benefits this sharing brought them. The intangible benefits they were less aware of.

In the course of time, through social, industrial, economic, educational, and scientific developments, communities became better organized. This allowed Man to feel and live more independently from his fellow man. Communal ties weakened.

All was fine. Everything which had been achieved by leaning together was now performed by hired hands. The benefits which were previously achieved through solidarity were still enjoyed, but the invisible benefits were missing. A few centuries passed. These were centuries lost to mankind. Finally some few people began to clear their perceptions and try to tell others about it. Most of them were burned or crucified.

Instead people sought the remedy in affluence, effort-saving inventions, education, recreation, gambling, dope, sexual follies, wars, and so on. Mankind has pursued these solutions to the point of exhaustion.

The love engendered by communal life and interdependence can be raised to the level of Cosmic Love. If Man develops an awareness of his true identity as a witness of the wholeness of God, the community he is part of attains its holistic shape, its integration in vertical and horizontal dimensions, spiritually, materially.

When Man reaches the Ultimate *Truth*, reaches direct communion or at-one-ment with God, what does his life look like? In this state of being, Man finds himself in full and tangible awareness of his oneness with the whole Universe. A deep sense of belonging to everything around him and everything around him belonging to him embraces him. A vibration of Agape Love quickens him and wipes away all kinds of psychic toxins. He becomes a man of Love. He becomes the Man described in the 13th chapter of the first Epistle to the Corinthians in the New Testament.

To attain this platform of awareness, we have to go through a process of training. The Abkhasian elect does it through Ahmusta Kebzeh, which includes a series of conscious breathing exercises under the meticulous coaching of a master. It is obvious that I cannot put down here the teaching of Kebzeh. But if anybody wants to know more about it, he may contact me freely through the publisher. For thousands and thousands of years, the message of this Kebzeh was given to hundreds of wisemen all over the world, and they applied it under various names in various parts of the world as they deemed proper according to the geographical, cultural, social, and vocational characteristics of their peoples. Ahmusta Kebzeh was given to Abraham, to Moses, to Buddha, to Zoroaster, to Jesus, and to Muhammed as the esoteric essence of the teachings of the religions these wisemen founded, and it was further applied to Islam to give birth to Islamic Sufism. However, our task in this book is not the teaching of spiritual development, but it is to point to its importance concerning the well-being of Man.

What I have explained can be summed up in a few words. To reach longevity, health and vigor and live life abundantly, the first thing we have to do is to get rid of the physical toxins and the psychological toxins in our system. The second thing we have to do is to acquire the right knowledge and guidance in order to use our now toxin-free being victoriously to reach abundant life. Remember, Jesus said: "I came that you might have life, and you might have it abundantly."

As I said before, try to get the *truth*, if you want to understand Abkhasian longevity; not only Abkhasians but *you* are eligible for it also, if you can get it.